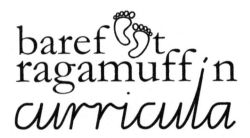

Copyright © 2013, 2015 by Kathy Jo DeVore. The eBook version may be printed for the use of one household and may not be resold. The print version may not be reproduced.

Table of Contents

Disclaimer 5

1. The Myth of the Caveman 7

2. Science and Politics 11

3. The Curse of the Mummy 15

4. The Digestive System: An Overview 19

5. What are Nutrients? 23

6. Industrial Food 29

7. Real Food 33

8. Fats, Part 1 37

9. Fats, Part 2 43

10. Protein, Part 1 47

11. Protein, Part 2 51

12. Lacto-Fermented Foods and Bone Broths 55

13. Dairy 59

14. Sweeteners 61

15. What are Anti-Nutrients? 65

16. Are Grains and Legumes All Bad All the Time? 69

17. A Low-Carb Lifestyle 73

18. Sleep and Play 77

A Few Recipes 81

Recommended Reading and Viewing 87

Works Cited 89

Disclaimer

Children, before reading this book, get permission from a parent or guardian.

To those parents and guardians:

This book goes against all conventional wisdom. Everything in it screams that the experts are wrong, that the way to good health is to be found by ignoring the majority of diet advice that you see from government officials and major health organizations. Because of this, it's in serious need of a disclaimer.

I am neither a medical professional nor a scientist. This book is, in essence, a research paper intended to explain nutrition from an ancestral health perspective to children. It is not intended to diagnose, treat, or prevent any sort of disease or health problem. It is for educational purposes only.

I make the following recommendations with the understanding that ultimately, you and you alone are responsible for what you choose to feed yourself and your family, and how you approach health for your family.

I highly recommend doing your own research and coming to your own conclusions about what constitutes a healthy diet. To that end, I have included suggested reading and viewing at the end of this book, all from an ancestral health perspective. Diet advice from a more conventional, government approved perspective is easy to find without my help.

For those with serious medical conditions, particularly those who are taking medication(s) for chronic health conditions, it is important that you speak to your doctor before changing your diet. Changes in diet can produce rapid changes in your health that could cause your medicine to harm rather than help you

1
The Myth of the Caveman

Long ago in the distant past, our ancestors—the cavemen—lived during the time period called the Paleolithic era. These cavemen were nomadic hunter-gatherers who spent their days traveling around, following the animals which they hunted for food and gathering wild edible plants. Cavemen were small and stupid, and they rarely lived past the age of 30-40 years old. Their short lives were full of hardship and hunger and endless toil. But lo, a discovery was made that ushered in a glorious new era, the Neolithic! This discovery was agriculture, and to it we owe our good health and our civilizations.

This is the way the story is usually taught, but it simply isn't true.

We can learn about cultures from the past in two ways. First, scientists called anthropologists study evidence about people and cultures that they find from long ago. Second, we can gain valuable insights into how hunter-gatherers of the past lived by studying modern hunter-gatherer cultures in the world today. And when we do these two things, quite a different picture of the cavemen begins to emerge.

Hardin Village and Indian Knoll

In Kentucky, the sites of two very different communities have been found and studied. Hardin Village existed about 500 years ago, and Indian Knoll existed about 3,000-5,000 years ago; a knoll is a small hill or mound. There were hundreds of skeletons found and studied from each location. This is very important. Think about it: If only a few skeletons were studied, it would be hard to know whether or not these were typical people of the time and area.

Imagine that there's a plane crash and ten people die. The wreck is never recovered. Sad, I know, but it's only pretend. Now imagine that anthropologists in the future found the site of this wreck. Seven of the skeletons were male and over six feet tall. They were in excellent health—you know, when they were alive. Two of the others were also male, shorter but still in excellent health. Only one skeleton was a woman. Would an anthropologist conclude from this evidence that people of our time period were generally in excellent health and very tall? Or that there were relatively few women in our society? Would he guess correctly that this was an unusual group, perhaps seven basketball players with two pilots and a flight attendant?

Hopefully, our anthropologist of the future would know that he needed to gather more information to form an accurate picture of the past. With a large sampling, we can get a better idea of what was normal among the population, and what was out of the ordinary. We can determine the average height and state of health and feel confident that the data—the information—is not merely a result of looking at an extreme like professional sports players. That's why it's important that both Hardin Village and Indian Knoll left behind so many skeletal remains.

Besides the skeletal remains, other evidence was also found that tells us something about the way these two groups of people lived. Anthropological evidence can include the tools the people used. Pottery used for making meals can sometimes still have residue from the food prepared on them!

So, what does the evidence from Hardin Village and Indian Knoll tell us?

Hardin Village was located in Eastern Kentucky and Indian Knoll was in Western Kentucky. Both areas had similar weather, water, plants, and animals. Neither group moved around much, if at all. We know that the people of Indian Knoll used the spear-thrower and the spear. The people of Hardin Village had pottery and permanent houses, and they used the bow and arrow.

These communities were very much alike, except in what they ate and how they came by their food. This is important because we cannot compare two groups who were too different. But when two groups are very similar in every way except for how they ate, then we can see that their differences in diet must have something to do with their differences in health.

The people of Hardin Village were farmers whose primary sources of food were corn, beans, and squash. They supplemented their mainly grain and legume diet with wild plants and nuts as well as meat from white-tailed deer, elk, raccoon, fox, wild turkey, and fish.

The people of Indian Knoll were hunter-gatherers whose primary source of food was meat. They hunted local white-tailed deer, raccoon, beaver, muskrat, otter, wild turkey, and box turtle. They fished and ate large quantities of mussels during times when they could be harvested. There is also evidence that the inhabitants collected wild fruits and nuts.

Which group do you think was the healthiest? The results may surprise you.

The overall life expectancy was lower at Hardin Village. That means that people died younger. Infant mortality was also higher for the Hardin Village farmers. That means that very young children were more likely to die from causes such as malnutrition—poor diet—and infectious diseases. Why would this be? People who are healthy are better able to fight off infectious diseases. Good health depends on getting proper nutrition.

The Hardin Village farmers had more cavities. The average was six or seven cavities per person, and even young children often had cavities. The Indian Knoll hunter-gatherers had an average of one or no cavities per person, and children under the age of twelve had no cavities at all.

Bone problems that indicate malnutrition were found among the Hardin Village farmers, but not the Indian Knoll hunter-gatherers.

The hunter-gatherers of Indian Knoll were healthier and lived longer lives than the farmers of Hardin Village.

As You Read this Book, Remember This…

Each one of us is responsible for his own decisions. No scientist, no teacher, no government official, and not even I will ever care about your health as much as you do. Your parents care almost as much as you because it hurts them to see you suffer. Still, if your health is poor, you're the one doing the suffering, and your parents aren't always around to tell you what to do. That's why it's in your best interest to understand what your food does as it goes through your digestive system, what it causes your body to do, and how it can make you sick. It's in your own best interest to understand the science and to use it to make wise decisions.

2

Science and Politics

In the late nineteen-sixties and through the seventies, the United States Senate, a branch of our government which makes laws, formed and maintained a committee to study hunger and malnutrition in the United States and determine what could be done about these issues. Malnutrition is a condition where a person does not get enough nutrients for good health. Senator McGovern led this committee, and eventually they released a report entitled "Dietary Goals of the United States," also known as the McGovern report. This report suggested that Americans should eat less fat, cholesterol, and refined sugars. Instead, they should eat more complex carbohydrates and fiber.

In the documentary Fat Head, Tom Naughton shows footage from a hearing regarding these recommendations. During this hearing, on July 26, 1977, Dr. Robert Olson said, "I pleaded in my report and will plead again orally here for more research on the problem before we make announcements to the American public." To this, Senator McGovern replied, "Well, I would only argue that senators don't have the luxury that a research scientist does of waiting until every last shred of evidence is in."

The Scientific Method

Do you know what the scientific method is? It's a set of techniques that scientists use to investigate observations and to acquire new knowledge.

The scientist begins by forming a hypothesis—a possible

explanation for a scientific problem. The next step is to experiment to test the hypothesis. To be valid, results must be consistent and repeatable. Repeatable means that another person could come along, perform the same experiment, and get the same results; consistent means that other research points towards the same conclusions. And finally, the scientist compares the results from the experiment with the hypothesis and forms a conclusion. Did the results support the hypothesis or disprove it? Did it lead to new observations that should be tested? If so, then more experiments may be necessary.

By continuing this process, we can learn more and more about our world and how things work. This process can also help us see how two events are related, whether we have a correlation or causation. A correlation is when two events are related, but neither causes the other to happen. For instance, more people drown when ice cream sales go up. Now, ice cream does not cause people to drown, so why do these things happen at the same time every year? The answer is simple: People buy more ice cream and swim more in the summer time when it's hot, and when people are swimming more, more people drown. There is no causation since neither causes the other; there is only correlation. To show causation, we need evidence which we can get from experimenting.

Do you remember Senator McGovern's reply to Dr. Olson? He said, "Well, I would only argue that senators don't have the luxury that a research scientist does of waiting until every last shred of evidence is in." I hope you can now see that waiting until the evidence is in is not a luxury. Without evidence, a hypothesis remains a hypothesis. It may be an observation. It may be someone's opinion. It may be a guess. But without evidence, it cannot be considered a fact, and it should never be a government recommendation.

USDA Dietary Guidelines

In time, the suggestions in the McGovern Report became the foundation for the USDA Dietary Guidelines. USDA stands for United States Department of Agriculture. In 1992, they introduced the Food Pyramid as an aid to understanding what we should eat. They periodically change the graphic representation of the guidelines, but the guidelines themselves have changed little—in spite of the evidence finally coming in and proving the guidelines wrong.

A man once told a man who worked for the USDA that their recommendations were wrong, that they actually made people sick. The USDA man laughed and said, "You're confused. There's another government organization that's responsible for people's health. It's called the Food and Drug Administration. We're the Department of Agriculture. Our job is to sell grains."

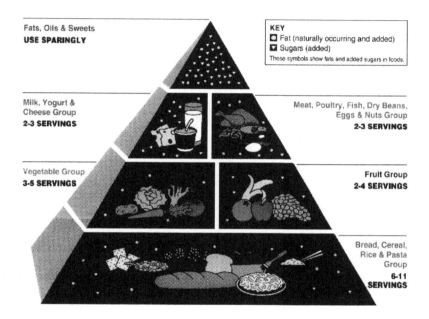

3

The Curse of the Mummy

Just like Hardin Village and Indian Knoll, the ancient Egyptians left plenty of bodies for modern scientists to study—mummies! Mummies are so well preserved that scientists can often even discover what the causes of death were, and what the overall state of health was before death. We also have written history from the Egyptians which describes how they lived and the types of medical problems they were experiencing.

Did you know that the ancient Egyptians ate exactly the kind of diet that is recommended by the USDA today? Ancient Egyptians lived along the fertile Nile River, an area with perfect conditions for growing food. The average Egyptian ate plenty of whole grain wheat and barley. During some periods, Egyptian soldiers were rationed five pounds of bread per day! Other foods common to the time were many varieties of fruits, vegetables, and nuts. Protein sources included fish and poultry. They ate almost no red meat. Instead of lard or tallow, which are animal fats, they used olive, sesame, and safflower oils for cooking. They used goat milk for drinking and making cheese, and they used honey instead of refined sugar or corn syrup.

According to the USDA recommendations, these people should have been in superb health, living long lives. And yet, they didn't. According to both the writings they left behind and the mummies, the ancient Egyptians suffered from the same types of problems we have today: obesity, heart disease, diabetes, and cavities, to name a few.

Other Peoples, Other Studies

During the 1930s, a dentist named Dr. Weston A. Price traveled throughout the world and observed groups of people who were untouched by what we call civilization, and the foods that come with it. These people still ate local, traditionally prepared foods. Although different groups ate different foods—there was no magic set of ingredients—they were free from the chronic diseases and cavities which plague western civilization. In fact, there is a long list of diseases which we now call the diseases of civilization because they do not appear in groups who eat local, traditional diets. It is only when these peoples come into contact with western society and begin to adopt a western diet that they become as ill as we have become.

In 2008, Gary Taubes published his book Good Calories, Bad Calories. In it, he discusses the many scientific studies that have been done over past. He discusses a number of scientists and doctors in addition to Dr. Price who met up with healthy, primitive peoples untouched by the chronic conditions we consider normal. These peoples, too, began to get sick when they adopted a western diet.

Gary Taubes also writes about Vilhjalmur Stefansson, an Arctic explorer who spent a decade among the Inuit. He returned to the lower states claiming that during this time, he'd eaten nothing but meat, mostly caribou with various amounts of fish, seal, polar bear, rabbits, birds, and eggs. This tale astounded scientists of his time. They believed that a person would die without a diet of many different kinds of food to give him all the vitamins and minerals necessary for good health. Stefansson and a Danish explorer, Karsten Anderson, became the subjects of a yearlong study in the winter of 1928. A team of a dozen people supervised the experiment. The team was made up of doctors, nutritionists, who are people who study nutrition, and anthropologists, who are people who study human societies. The study started by evaluating the health of the men. Stefansson and Anderson ate nothing but meat for the whole year, many different kinds of meat. At the end of the year, the two men were healthier than they had been at the beginning of the year (324).

What Does All of This Have to Do with Cavemen?

Just as anthropologists can tell us about the health problems of ancient Egyptians, they can also tell us about the health of hunter-gatherer groups around the world and throughout history. In fact, it's said that just by looking at skeletal remains, an anthropologist can tell whether the person was a hunter-gatherer or a farmer in life. Like the Indian-Knoll hunter-gatherers mentioned in the first chapter, hunter-gatherer groups are healthier as a whole. They show fewer signs of cavities and bone problems due to malnutrition.

Because of this, some people decided to go way back in time for their diet advice, all the way to the Paleolithic Era when there were no farmers, only hunter-gatherers—cavemen. This way of eating is called primal, paleo, or sometimes, the caveman diet.

The idea is simple: Since this is the way people ate for most of human history, and people were actually healthier prior to agriculture, we should model our diets after theirs. Many different people have written books about this way of eating, and each author's view of the diet is slightly different. The common belief that joins them all is that we are made to eat certain foods. Those foods keep us healthy. Other foods make us sick.

All of these ideas together are sometimes called Ancestral Health. That means we're looking to the past to know how to stay healthy today. We can't become true hunter-gatherers in modern America, but we can surely improve on the Standard American Diet which is making us all so sick and fat.

Our mascot Cro will appear at the end of each chapter to give the cave perspective on the chapter's topic.

The Digestive System: An Overview

What does your body do with the food you eat?

Digestion is the process of breaking down food for your body to use. Your body uses food at a cellular level. That means each tiny, microscopic cell takes nutrients from your food to perform its tasks—muscle cells to move, lung cells to process oxygen, and blood cells to move it all around the body.

Your digestive system starts in your mouth. The act of chewing breaks food down into small pieces before you swallow it. The saliva, or spit, in your mouth helps to break down chemicals in your food. When you swallow, food travels down your esophagus to your stomach.

The stomach is a stretchy sack. It churns the food and mixes the food with gastric juices, also called stomach acid, to continue breaking it down into a liquid mixture. Gastric juices also helps kill germs that might otherwise make us ill. Then, the stomach slowly releases this mixture into the small intestine.

The small intestine is a long tube. How long? It's about twenty-two feet long. That's as long as a small bus or a large van! Its diameter, the width of the tube, is only 1 ½ to 2 inches. While food is in the small intestine, three organs help to break down the food even further—the pancreas, the liver, and the gallbladder. The pancreas releases enzymes, substances which break down food, and it also releases insulin, a hormone which controls blood sugar. The liver releases bile, which helps the body absorb fat. And the gallbladder stores the bile until the body needs it.

In the small intestine, the body begins to absorb the food. Tiny finger-like projections in the small intestine called villi soak up nutrients from food, absorbing the nutrients as the food travels through the digestive tract. From there, nutrients are sent throughout the entire body in the blood.

The large intestine is another tube, this one about 3-4 inches wide and about five feet long. The body has absorbed most of the nutrients by the time the food gets to the large intestine, also called the bowels. What's left over is waste material that your body won't use, also known as poop. From here, it's toilet time.

The Urinary System

You may be wondering about pee. The digestive system does not produce pee; the urinary system does.

The urinary tract is made up of the kidneys, which are the organs which filter blood, the ureters, which are tubes that transfer pee from the kidneys to the bladder, which is a stretchy bag that holds urine until you feel the urge to go pee. Urine, or pee, exits the body through the urethra.

When the kidneys filter the blood, they send water, nutrients, protein, and glucose back into the bloodstream. They remove waste products like excess water, urea, which is produced when your body breaks down protein, urochrome, which is a colored blood product that makes urine yellow, salts, creatinine, which is produced from the normal breakdown of muscle, byproducts of bile from the liver, and ammonia.

Filtered blood goes back to the bloodstream. What's left over is a yellowish liquid called urine or pee. A liter of blood passes through the kidneys every minute. The kidneys clean all of the blood in our bodies about once an hour. Adults produce 1-2 liters of pee per day.

What Would Cro Think?

It's likely that Cro did not know a lot about how his digestive and urinary systems worked. But I bet he did know that when food made him sick, he shouldn't eat that food anymore. For Cro, though, this was probably easier to figure out. Since his diet came from hunting and gathering, it was constantly changing. When it came to plants, he ate the foods that were growing right then, and they'd only be available for a short time. Our grocery stores today carry the same foods almost all year long. When we eat the same foods all the time, we may think sick is normal.

5

What are nutrients?

Nutrients are substances necessary for growth, metabolism, and other functions of the body. Metabolism is the process of burning some of these nutrients for energy. When we talk about food, we discuss how many calories various foods have. Calories are the basic unit of energy found in foods. The more calories a food has, the more energy it provides.

When we discuss nutrition, there are two types of nutrients that must be explained: micronutrients and macronutrients.

Micronutrients

The prefix "micro" is from the Greek and means "small." Micronutrients are nutrients that we need in small amounts to help the body grow, develop, and stay healthy. The two kinds of micronutrients are vitamins and minerals. Vitamins are organic substances, which means that they contain carbon and come from living things. Minerals are inorganic substances, which means that they do not contain carbon or come from living things.

Many different types of vitamins and minerals are needed because they play different roles in the body. Vitamin D, which is necessary for bone health, can be produced by your body when you get out in the sun, but most other vitamins need to come from our food. Vitamin A is necessary for strong eyes, vitamin C supports the immune system, and the B vitamins help the body produce protein and energy. A variety of minerals is also needed, such as calcium for bone and tooth health, iron for transporting oxygen throughout the body, and zinc for supporting the immune system.

Minerals have other functions, too. They are required for some enzymes to work. That means without minerals, many of the chemical reactions which take place in the body would not happen. Also, when minerals dissolve in water, they break into ions. Ions are atoms or molecules that do not have an equal number of electrons, which have a negative charge, and protons, which have a positive charge. That means that ions have either a negative or positive charge, depending on whether they have an extra electron or an extra proton. Ions formed in body fluids are called electrolytes. Electrolytes such as sodium, potassium, and chloride, help control the movement of water in and out of cells.

People can now buy bottles of vitamins and minerals at the grocery store, but these micronutrients are not as good as getting them from real food for a number of reasons. Did you notice that some of those vitamins and minerals mentioned above had the same jobs? That's because they work together to keep you healthy. Vitamins and minerals often work together synergistically; that means that together, they have a much greater effect than they have alone. Vitamins and minerals which work together are often found together in foods. Vitamins and minerals that require fat to be absorbed by the body are found in foods with the necessary amount of fat.

These relationships are complex. When scientists attempt to simplify the body's need for micronutrients to a recommended amount to be taken daily, created in a lab instead of found in nature, they miss the point. Proper nutrition begins and ends with proper food, not labeled jars.

Macronutrients

The prefix "macro" is from the Greek and means "big" or "large." Macronutrients are nutrients that we need in large amounts. They are literally the building blocks of the food we eat, and as such, they provide calories for energy. The three broad classes of macronutrients are fat, protein, and carbohydrate.

Fat

Fat is necessary for life. Without it, we die. So, what does fat do that's so important?

Our bodies use fats for maintaining cell membranes, promoting growth and development, and carrying essential vitamins through the blood stream. Our brains are mostly fat, about 60% by weight. Too little fat in the diet has also been linked to depression.

One gram of fat has nine calories, which means that fat provides more than twice as much energy as the other macronutrients. It makes us feel full for longer, which means we don't feel the need to eat as often. Fat also makes food taste better.

Protein

Our bodies use proteins for growing and repairing tissues, building muscle, supporting our immune systems, and producing enzymes and hormones which are necessary for our bodies to work properly. Enzymes are special proteins in living things that control chemical reactions. Hormones are messenger chemicals that cause a specific response in cells and tissues. Like fat, protein is necessary for life.

Carbohydrate

Carbohydrate heavy foods make up the base of the USDA food pyramid.

As we digest carbohydrates, they break down into glucose, a form of sugar. Table sugar is made up of about half glucose and half fructose. People who eat according to the USDA food pyramid get most of their energy from carbohydrates. That means that they literally get most of their energy from sugar.

Unlike fat and protein, carbohydrates are not necessary for life.

Carbohydrates as Brain Food

Many people say that our brains require glucose to function. Because of this, these people, including the USDA, recommend that most of our calories come from carbohydrates. However, when we avoid carbohydrates in our diets, our bodies can use protein and fat to make glucose to support brain functions. This process is called gluconeogenesis, and it uses amino acids from protein and glycerol from fat. Our bodies can make the amount of glucose that our brains need, so there's no reason to get that glucose from our diets.

Glucose is also not the only brain food. Fatty acids are broken down into pieces in the liver, forming ketone bodies. These ketones can then be used by both the body and the brain for energy.

Macronutrients and Insulin

Fats have more calories than proteins and carbohydrates. Each gram of fat has nine calories. By comparison, each gram of protein or carbohydrate has only four calories. Because of this, many people think that fats make people fat. They think that a diet high in fat will have too many calories, and that if all of that energy is not used through activity and exercise, it will be stored as fat. It also seems to make sense that fat would cause fat. However, the body requires a hormone called insulin to store fat, and the body doesn't send out insulin when we eat fat.

So what causes the body to produce insulin? Our bodies produce insulin to deal with excess glucose in our blood, what we call blood sugar. If our blood sugar gets too high, we die. The pancreas sends insulin out to lower blood sugar. One way it does this is by storing the excess glucose as fat. Our body uses fat to store energy to use between meals. If our bodies didn't store some fat, then we'd have to keep eating almost constantly to maintain energy. We would have a difficult time sleeping without starving to death. But storing too much fat is not healthy.

Do you remember which macronutrient breaks down into glucose when it's digested? Carbohydrates do. Protein raises insulin in the blood a little, but carbohydrates raise it by large amounts. And when insulin is high, the body stores those calories as fat.

Of the three macronutrients, carbohydrate is the only one which is not essential for life. Remember Stefansson, Anderson, and the Inuit. Without fat and protein, people would get sick and die quickly. Without carbohydrates, people have been known to become healthier.

Carbohydrate and Vitamins

The supervisors of the experiment on Stefansson and Anderson felt that if the men only ate meat, they would get sick because of vitamin deficiencies. A vitamin deficiency is when the body does not get enough of a vitamin. Remember that vitamins help support various systems in the body like the immune system, so a vitamin deficiency can be deadly. But that never happened; the men didn't develop vitamin deficiencies.

In Good Calories, Bad Calories, Gary Taubes reports that years after the experiment, nutritionists would establish that eating lots of carbohydrates uses up the body's supply of B vitamins; the body needs more of them when a high carbohydrate diet is eaten. Theodore Van Itallie testified this in 1973 in front of Senator McGovern's Select Committee. A similar argument is being made today concerning vitamin C. It seems that glucose makes it harder for your body's cells to take-up vitamin C (325).

Why is this important? Many people think that grains are an important part of the diet because of the vitamins they have. But grains are extremely high in carbohydrate, so even though they have vitamins, they may also cause your body to need more vitamins. They are also packed with anti-nutrients which make it difficult for our bodies to use the vitamins that they do possess. We'll talk about anti-nutrients in a later chapter.

What Would Cro Think?

Cro would have eaten lots of different foods. He couldn't just eat his favorite foods all the time. His favorite animal foods relied on finding the animal and having a successful hunt. His favorite plant foods depended on them being in season. In season means the time when the plants are producing food. For instance, some types of berry bushes produce berries only during the summer months. There would be none of those berries to be found in the spring, fall, or winter. Different foods have different types of nutrients, so that kind of variety in the diet helped Cro to get plenty of nutrients.

6

Industrial Food

In today's modern world, the grocery store is a scary place. That may sound funny, but there are items on the shelves that people a few generations ago wouldn't have recognized as food at all, items filled with ingredients created in a lab instead of found in nature.

Look at nature. In nature, we find diversity. Large grazing animals live side-by-side with birds, and all of these animals are healthier because of it. Different plants grow together. Symbiotic relationships form. A symbiotic relationship is one in which different species act in ways that benefit each other as well as themselves. Birds eat the bugs that large grazing animals uncover as they walk through the grass. They benefit the grazers by eating the bugs that bite and annoy the them. The birds also peck at manure from the grazers to get bits of undigested food and bug larvae. In the process of doing this, they spread the manure, which fertilizes the land that helps to feed them all.

A healthy farm imitates nature in this diversity. Chickens perform the same tasks for sheep, goats, and cattle that birds in the wild do for grazing animals. Of course, local wild birds chip in to help, too. We had a pig who would lie still while sparrows came and groomed him every morning. Their benefit was food, and his was comfort. The farm always benefits from multiple species interacting, and all the species benefit from the fresh air, sunshine, and natural diet. On a well run farm, there is no waste. Food and milk that the family doesn't eat will go to chickens, rabbits, and pigs. Manure from the animals fertilizes the garden, and the garden feeds the family and the animals.

Contrast this with modern industrial farms. On these farms, there is no diversity. There are chicken farms which cram chickens together in small spaces with no room to move, and no sunshine, in buildings where workers need gas masks to enter. There are feed lots where cattle are in conditions so disgusting that they need medicine in their food every day just to keep them alive. There are fields with acre after acre of corn or soy beans which will be processed and turned into those scary packages on grocery store shelves. These farms do produce waste. We call it pollution, and it affects the land and the water, not just on those farms, but in the surrounding areas as well.

These reasons would be enough to be against industrial farming. However, it also turns out that the food they are creating is not as healthy as more naturally grown food. Food is only as safe and healthy as the environment in which it is grown. We'll talk more about this in chapters to come.

What is Industrial Food?

Industrial food is created by industrial processes. Many different practices create industrial food.

Consider corn syrup. Have you ever eaten corn and thought to yourself, "Wow! That tastes just like sugar!" Of course not. Some corn is mildly sweet, but not in the same way that sugar or honey is sweet. So how does corn become super sweet corn syrup?

Corn becomes corn syrup through an industrial process. Corn is broken down and separated into different products. Remember that during digestion, the body uses enzymes to digest food. Also remember that carbohydrates easily break down into glucose—sugar—during digestion. To make corn syrup, companies use enzymes to predigest one of the corn products to break it down into sugar.

Other grains, as well as legumes like soy beans, also go through a number of processes which break them down and change their forms. Because they are inexpensive to buy, they are added to many things as filler. Consider this: If corn syrup is cheaper to produce than meat, then a company can make more money by using corn syrup as an ingredient in sausage. That's what a filler is, something to take the place of better ingredients in order to produce more of a product for a cheaper price.

This type of food is often called processed food because of the processes it goes through before it's sent to stores. Other processes remove fats from food to make it last longer on store shelves without going bad. Ultra-pasteurized milk products work under the same principle—not health, but shelf-life. Shelf-life is the amount of time that a product can sit on a store shelf without going bad. Vegetables can go bad within days, and milk can go bad within weeks, but it's a longstanding joke that those puffy yellow pastries with the cream filling will still look and taste the same in twenty years or more.

Frankenfood

In the book Frankenstein, a scientist creates a monster and brings it to life. We use the word Frankenfood because, like the creature in the book, some foods on your grocery store shelves have been tampered with by well-meaning scientists who created something potentially monstrous.

Throughout the history of agriculture, farmers have tried different practices to get more food and a better quality of food. For instance, if a farmer has some sort of problem in his garden, but one plant does better than all the other plants while this problem continues, he might take the seed from that plant to use the next year. From then on, his seeds will be the descendants of that plant. This is a good thing that can help produce plants that are naturally more drought tolerant or pest resistant. Farmers have also done things like plant two or more kinds of plants together—called companion planting—to help the plants to thrive. For example, if the farmer plants broccoli with the herb rosemary and geranium flowers, the rosemary and geraniums both protect the broccoli against insects which harm the plant. These are safe practices which help and do no harm.

Frankenfood is food that has been genetically modified in a lab. Genes are units of heredity. We—all life forms—get them from our parents, and we pass them on to our offspring. In people, genes determine physical characteristics like eye color, and they also tell about what types of health problems we're likely to have. That's why doctors often want to know what health problems your family members have had.

Genes also determine characteristics in plants, which is why a farmer will save seed from the best of his plants, the ones which produce the best vegetables and are the most drought tolerant and pest resistant.

Genetically modified means that scientists have changed the genes in a plant. In some cases, food has been modified to not die when a certain type of poison is sprayed on it. That way, agriculturists can spray an entire field with poisons to kill weeds without killing the crop. Other foods have been modified to produce more food, or to have a chemical in them that's believed by scientists to be healthy. This is sometimes done by adding genes from other plants or even animals to a plant.

Are these plants now dangerous? The problem is that we don't know. Scientists have radically changed the very genes in our food. Would a squash with animal genes still truly be a squash? Could it have a different effect on our bodies than a squash that wasn't genetically modified? The truth is that we don't know the answer to these questions yet.

What Would Cro Think?

Cro never ate a single food that had been genetically modified, that had been sprayed with poisons, or that had been predigested in a factory. He ate foods directly from Nature. Nature doesn't produce pollution, and we can avoid most pollution when we imitate Nature instead of trying to do things in the cheapest, easiest way possible. I bet Cro might want to know why we think something is cheaper and easier when it harms the land we rely on for life.

7

Real Food

So what is real food?

Real food is food in its most natural, healthful state, food that hasn't been tampered with and processed to the point where it would not have been recognizable as food a few generations ago. Real food is full of vitamins and minerals, and essential fats and proteins. I would also argue that real food is grown and raised in safe, natural environments. People don't get sick when visiting a real food farm, and they don't need any special protective gear, either.

Real food is whole food. Remember the discussion in the last chapter about industrial foods? In industrial foods, grains and soy beans are often broken down into different products. These products are then put back together in different ways and added to actual foods to produce the boxes and bags on grocery store shelves.

Whole food is different. It's not broken down into different products to be used as additives and fillers. Instead, whole foods consist of the whole, edible portion of a food.

Our bodies need other nutrients in order to use many vitamins and minerals. Without the other nutrients, those much needed vitamins and minerals go straight through the digestive tract and into the toilet. But remember: Whole foods have vitamins and minerals combined with the other nutrients that they need to be absorbed by our bodies.

This synergy—the way nutrients work together—is what is missing in industrial food. Food is more than the sum of its parts. We can't merely add a bunch of vitamins to a food, or take a vitamin pill every day, and expect to be healthy. Our bodies cannot use these nutrients in isolation like that. Sometimes, in fact, vitamins that would be good for us become potentially dangerous when they're taken in isolation. The body can't use them in this way, but it will still store some of them. These vitamins can build up in the body until they cause harm. The results of many studies have suggested that some vitamins are dangerous if we take too much of them, but researchers always seem to study synthetic vitamins in isolation instead of natural vitamins as part of a whole food diet.

What is Organic Food?

Many people believe that organic food is food that hasn't been treated with all of the chemicals used on conventional food. Sadly, this is not always the case.

Organic food has a legal definition, a list of requirements that must be met in order to be called organic. You've probably seen the phrase certified organic. That means that a group oversees the farmer to make sure he only uses approved chemicals.

You see, it is true that organic foods cannot be grown with conventional chemicals, but that does not mean that organic foods are grown without chemicals, even poisonous chemicals. There are many chemicals which have been approved for growing foods organically.

If chemicals can be used on organic foods, then what makes them different than conventionally grown food? The difference is that organic chemicals are from natural sources. Conventional herbicides, which are poisons that kill weeds, and pesticides, which are poisons that kill insects, can be synthetic. Synthetic means that they're man-made instead of found in nature. Because they are found in nature, organically approved chemicals may be better for the environment, but not necessarily.

Are organic foods no better than conventional ones? In the end, it depends on the organic farm in question. Some of them are producing high quality, highly nutritious food in ways that are good for the planet. With others, it's the same as conventional farming with organically approved chemicals.

Local, Sustainable Food

Local, sustainable agriculture may or may not be certified organic, and it may or may not use chemicals. The beauty of local food is that you can know your farmer. You can probably visit his farm, see how he does things, and ask questions.

Local food also supports local economy, which means how money is spent in your community. Think about this. Did you know that many vegetables in your local grocery store were grown in foreign countries? When people buy vegetables grown in China, the money leaves your local community, even your country, and goes somewhere else. But when you buy from a local farmer, the money stays in your community. That means the farmer has money to spend at local stores, and the people of those stores have more money to spend. The economy of the community is healthier.

Another problem with non-local food is that of shipping. Can you imagine the resources necessary to ship food all the way around the world? Think of just your own town or city. How many ships does it take to bring food around the world to feed your town for a month? For a year? How many trucks does it take to get the food to the stores? Now consider that there are about 20,000 towns and cities in the United States.

Sustainable means a system that can keep on going. Conventional farming and organic farming that require chemicals are not sustainable. Without the chemicals, the farming stops. Worse, applying all of these chemicals hurts both the land and us. Just as we get nutrients from the food we eat, plants get many of their nutrients from the soil. So what happens to the plants when they're grown in sick soil and chemical fertilizers, covered in poisons to prevent weeds and pests? We get plants which lack nutrients. Plants that lack nutrients lead to people who lack nutrients. And just as the plants take up poisons from the land, we take up poisons from the plants.

Sustainable farming is different. Remember the discussion in the previous chapter about diversity in nature and farming? Sustainable farming improves the land by fertilizing with manure. The bodies of animals, and people, are not 100% efficient at removing nutrients from the food we eat. When animal manure is returned to the land, so are all of those unused nutrients, as well as other chemicals that plants need to thrive. Manure can be composted along with other products such as paper and rotten food. Composting turns what others consider trash and waste into healthy soil. Composting can even break down some chemicals which are harmful to the environment and make them safe again.

The goal of sustainable farming is to farm in a way that improves the land, leaving it better, healthier, than it was before, without needing to bring in materials from outside the farm.

What Would Cro Think?

For Cro, local, sustainable food was the only option. His community was small, made up of people who were his friends and family, and they all worked together. Today, our communities are large. Most of us can't possibly know all of the people who live in our towns. That makes it hard to care about our communities as much as Cro would have cared about his, but that doesn't mean we can't try.

8

Fats, Part 1

Fat is my favorite macro-nutrient, and it's my belief that fat is where we should get most of our calories. Have you heard people talk about eating a low calorie diet? It's easier to eat fewer calories when you eat lots of fat. That's because fat makes you feel full and satisfied, so you don't need to eat as much of it. And remember, fat doesn't raise insulin. That means that even if you eat a lot of fat, your insulin won't spike, or go up high. Protein raises insulin a little, and carbohydrates raises insulin a lot. So, if you want to keep your insulin normal—and you should—then the best thing to do is to eat a high fat, moderate protein, low carbohydrate diet.

Fats are a major source of energy, especially for people who don't eat many carbohydrates. Fats are also called triglycerides because they are a combination of three fatty acid molecules and one glycerol molecule. During digestion, fats are absorbed through the walls of the small intestine. The glycerol is separated from the fatty acids. The fatty acids are broken down into pieces in the liver, forming ketone bodies. These ketones can then be used by the body for energy.

Some of the fatty acids are called essential fatty acids. Our bodies cannot produce them, but they are necessary for life. We must get them from the foods we eat.

Fats also help the body to absorb fat-soluble vitamins like A, D, E, and K. Fat-soluble means that they dissolve in fat, not water. Without enough fat, our bodies can't use these vitamins even if we get plenty of them in our diets!

Like all real food, healthy fats come from natural sources.

The Omegas

Omega-3 and omega-6 fatty acids are the two groups of essential fatty acids. Both of them are absolutely necessary. However, our body needs them in a specific ratio. A ratio is a specific amount of each. Our bodies need them in balance, 1 omega-3 fatty acid for every 1 omega-6 fatty acid.

The problem is that omega-6 fatty acids are high in foods like grain and corn. They're also high in animals that eat grain and corn. That means that if we eat these foods, we can have too many omega-6 fatty acids. Many Americans have diets that have ratios of 35:1. That means that they eat 35 omega-6 fatty acids for every 1 omega-3 fatty acid.

Many people take a supplement to get more omega-3 fatty acids into their diets. A supplement is something to take to make up for a deficiency. When people don't get enough omega-3 fatty acids, or vitamins or minerals, they take supplements.

To balance out our omega-3 to omega-6 ratio, we can also eat foods with less omega-6 fatty acids and more omega-3 fatty acids. Grass-fed meat, which we'll talk about in one of the protein chapters, has more omega-3 fatty acids than meat from grain fed animals. Fish and nuts are also good sources of omega-3 fatty acids.

Saturated Fats

Have you heard the terms saturated and unsaturated fats and wondered what the difference is? The difference has to do with how the molecules bond, or connect together. Each type of fat is made up of a triglyceride and three long chains of hydrocarbons. Hydrocarbons are made up entirely of hydrogen and carbon. Saturated fats only have single bonds in the hydrocarbon chains. These chains are evenly filled, or saturated, with hydrogen. Unsaturated fats have double bonds. The double bonds replace hydrogen, so they are not saturated, or unsaturated.

You may have noticed something about how saturated and unsaturated fats are different. Saturated fats are solid, or near solid, at room temperature, and unsaturated fats are liquid. Room temperature is considered to be between 68 and 77° F. Some saturated fats need cooler temperatures to become solid.

Saturated fats include fats from animal sources, such as eggs, meat, bone marrow, and organ meats, and full fat dairy products like butter, cheese, cream, and sour cream. Coconuts and avocados also have saturated fat. We can gain the benefits from eating saturated fats by eating the whole foods, but we can also use just the fats.

Fats from meats that are made to cook in are called tallow or lard. Tallow comes from beef or lamb while lard comes from pigs. There are also poultry fats which can come from chickens, ducks, or geese.

Butter is flavorful, but when people cook with it, sometimes it burns. Some people like to use ghee instead. Ghee is butter that's been cooked and had the milk solids removed. It doesn't have to be refrigerated, and it doesn't burn like butter.

Coconut oil has many health benefits. It contains lauric acid, which boosts the immune system. It's anti-viral, anti-bacterial, and anti-fungal. That means it can destroy microbes that might otherwise harm you. Coconut oil can also protect the body against some toxins.

Avocado oil is good for cooking at low temperatures. It's also good for making homemade salad dressings.

Unsaturated Fats

Many nuts are good sources of unsaturated fats. Almonds, pistachios, walnuts, macadamias, pecans, and hazelnuts, to name a few, all contain healthy unsaturated fats.

Healthy unsaturated fats are also found in olive and sesame oils, and nut oils such as walnut and macadamia. They are not good for cooking since they shouldn't be heated to high temperatures. When they are heated, they break down and form free radicals, which will be explained in the next chapter.

In Get Your Fats Straight, Sarah Pope says that sesame oil is the exception to the no-cooking rule. Raw sesame seed oil—not toasted sesame seed oil—has antioxidants which are activated when it's heated (Chapter 10).

But just because a fat is natural, that doesn't make it healthy. Oils like grapeseed and hemp seed are high in omega-6 fatty acids, making them poor choices of fat in the diet. Flaxseed oil is high in omega-3 fatty acids, but it also has phytoestrogen. Phytoestrogen is a compound similar to the human sex hormone estrogen. Because of this, use of flaxseed oil should be limited.

How Important is Fat?

In the "all-meat" diet of Arctic explorers Stefansson and Anderson, about 80% of their calories came from fat! Stefansson wrote an article about his experiences, "Adventures in Diet," which appeared the November 1935 issue of Harper's Monthly Magazine. In it, he said that the only problems they had were when the overseers of the experiment kept them on lean meat instead of fatty meat. He compared it to eating half-starved caribou in the Arctic when food was short. He described his symptoms as, "diarrhea and a feeling of general baffling discomfort."

But what about heart disease? Isn't it dangerous to eat that much fat? Actually, there are no studies that prove that saturated fat causes heart disease, heart attacks, or any health problem at all. At the beginning of this book, we talked about how the government made recommendations before all the facts were in—Senator McGovern stated this himself.

There was a study that showed that when rabbits are fed cholesterol, they have more heart attacks. Cholesterol is a substance in saturated fats which we'll discuss in the next chapter. The problem here is that rabbits are herbivores. Their natural diet has no cholesterol in it.

There were studies that showed correlation, not causation, between fat and heat disease. Some studies, in fact, only used part of the data available to form their conclusions. The most famous of these is Ancel Keys' Seven Countries Study. His conclusions were based on data from seven countries, but he actually had data from twenty-two countries.

People began to believe that fat causes heart disease, but no study ever proved it. In fact, some researchers and science writers today are baffled because new studies are showing that some fats lower the risk of heart disease and other health problems. Because they already believe that fat is the bad macronutrient, they often ignore or downplay evidence to the contrary. They assume that something weird is going on. They "know" that fat is bad, and it never occurs to them that they might be wrong, or to look more closely at the researched that "proved" fat is bad.

What Would Cro Think?

Like Stefansson and Anderson, Cro would have recognized that the best meats were the fatty ones. He would have enjoyed fats anywhere he could find them. Just like us, Cro would have felt full and satisfied when he ate lots of fat. In times of food shortage, when eating too many half-starved animals, he would have been less satisfied. He might have even gotten depressed until his diet improved again.

9

Fats, Part 2

Industrial Oils

Industrial oils include oils made from grains, soybeans, corn, and peanuts. These foods shouldn't be eaten, and neither should the fats from them. Canola and vegetable oils, which are often recommended by the government and major health organizations, are also industrial oils which should be avoided.

Industrial oils are often rancid as soon as they're removed from the plant material. A rancid oil is one that smells and tastes bad. Rancid oils also contain free radicals. Free radicals are molecules that can damage cells in the body. To understand how free radicals do damage, you need to know a little bit about atoms and molecules. A free radical is an atom or molecule which has an unpaired electron. Electrons don't want to be unpaired. A free radical can damage cells by robbing cell molecules of their electrons. The new, damaged molecule is now missing an electron, making it a free radical, too.

Antioxidants are molecules that prevent free radicals from harming cells. Many vitamins are antioxidants, such as vitamins A, C, and E. It's best to get them through whole food because the body can more easily absorb them from a whole food source.

Hydrogenated and Trans Fats

Fats are hydrogenated to make unsaturated fats solid at room temperature. Manufacturers change the fat by adding hydrogen molecules to it. Many people believe that saturated fats are bad for us, so they tried to make unsaturated fats that acted like saturated fats. Hydrogenation also gives the oils a longer shelf-life. Trans fatty acids are created during this process.

Hydrogenation damages the fat, making it unsafe to eat.

What About Cholesterol?

Cholesterol is a waxy substance needed for building and repairing cells. Many high fat foods are high in cholesterol.

Many doctors and scientists today tell people to watch their cholesterol. That means that they're not supposed to let the cholesterol in their blood get too high, and that they should avoid foods that are high in cholesterol. They say this because they believe that people with high cholesterol are more likely to develop heart disease.

Is this true? Should we watch our cholesterol and avoid foods with cholesterol?

It is true that people with high cholesterol may develop other problems such as heart disease as well. High cholesterol isn't the cause, though. It's one of the symptoms. Remember when we talked about correlation? A correlation is when two things happen at the same time, but neither causes the other. Cholesterol does not cause heart disease or any other health problem, but there is a correlation between high cholesterol and other health problems.

In fact, cholesterol is so important to your health that every cell in your body can make it. That's right, your body makes cholesterol. Cholesterol is necessary for building and repairing cells.

So what causes high cholesterol? The same thing that causes the diseases of civilization—high carbohydrate diets.

Statins are medicines that reduce cholesterol. If the scientists who say that high cholesterol causes heart disease are right, then reducing cholesterol should prevent or cure heart disease, right? But they do not. There's never been a single study that proved that taking statins will cure heart disease or prevent heart attacks.

And consider this: Many prescription drugs have side effects. Side effects are problems that a drug can cause while trying to help a medical problem. One of the side effects people have from taking statins is muscle weakness.

Do you know what kind of cells your heart is made of? Muscle cells! Your heart is a large muscle that pumps day and night to send blood throughout your body. It seems to me that taking medicine that weakens muscles can't possibly be good for your heart.

What Would Cro Think?

Cro would not have cared about cholesterol. It's in plenty of his favorite foods, and his body needed it as much as yours, but no one ever worried about cholesterol until this century. He also would not have recognized plants like corn and rapeseed as places to get fat. Can you imagine squeezing corn hard enough to get oil out of corn? Cro could not, either. It requires an industrial process to get oil out of corn.

10

Protein, Part 1

Proteins are chains of molecules called amino acids. Amino acids link together to form different types of proteins. Your body needs twenty different amino acids to build proteins. The body can make eleven of these, but nine of them are essential. Essential amino acids are ones that we must get from our food. Complete proteins contain all of the amino acids in the correct amounts. Incomplete proteins lack some of the amino acids that we need. Animal products are the best sources from complete proteins.

Happy animals taste better. While some people believe that it's wrong to consume meat, we believe that it's wrong to consume animals which were raised in misery and in horrific conditions just so we can get our daily protein. The old ways of raising animals are best, not just for the animals, but also for us.

And that daily allotment of protein is important. The body cannot store protein or amino acids for later use, so we need to eat protein regularly. Every cell in your body contains protein. Our bodies use protein for growing and repairing tissues, building muscle, supporting the immune system, and producing enzymes and hormones which are necessary for our bodies to work properly. Protein is necessary for life. Without it, we die.

It is also a simple fact that there are some nutrients which can only be obtained naturally through animal products. Amino acids are the building blocks of proteins. While we can get some amino acids through plant sources, meat and fish are complete proteins; they contain all of the amino acids necessary for life.

Vitamin A is important for normal vision. It supports the immune and reproductive systems, and it also helps the heart, lungs, kidneys, and other organs to work properly. True vitamin A can be found only in meat, egg yolks, dairy, and fish. Orange and green vegetables have beta carotene. The body can convert beta carotene into vitamin A, but it is not vitamin A itself, and the body needs six times as much beta carotene as true vitamin A.

Vitamin B12 maintains nerve and blood cells. It's necessary for making DNA, found in every cell in the body, and for normal functioning of the brain. Top sources for vitamin B12 are shellfish, liver, fish eggs, octopus, fish, crab and lobster, beef, lamb, cheese, and eggs.

Vitamin D helps the body to use the mineral calcium, which is important for bone health, and the mineral phosphorus, which is important for using protein. Our bodies can produce vitamin D if we get enough sunlight. Fair skinned individuals produce more vitamin D in a shorter amount of time than dark skinned individuals. This is because the same pigments which protect a dark skinned person from the sun also block vitamin D production. Not everyone gets enough sunlight to produce adequate vitamin D. Food sources include shrimp, wild salmon, sardines, full-fat dairy, and egg yolks.

Zinc is necessary for growth and development, for supporting the immune and reproductive systems, and for healthy brain function. Zinc is found in red meat. While zinc can be found in grains and legumes, so can anti-nutrients. Anti-nutrients prevent the body from using the nutrients in foods, and they can even rob your body of nutrients from other foods. It's much easier for the body to digest and absorb zinc from red meat sources.

Grass-Fed Meat

Industrial meat is raised on corn, soy beans, and sometimes, animal parts. That's a problem, particularly with cattle. Cows were made to eat grass, not grains and legumes, and certainly not other cows.

Over the years, there have been more and more reports of e. coli, a common bacteria that can make people sick. Industrial meat is the cause. A cow's stomach is not naturally a very acidic place. Grass-fed cows have some e. coli in their guts, but it doesn't affect us. Why? It doesn't affect us because our stomachs are naturally very acidic places. E. coli that survives in a grass-fed cow's gut dies when it enters ours.

Something happens to the gut of a cow fed grains and legumes, though. The cow's gut becomes more acidic, like ours. This kills all the normal e. coli. But there are always some which survive. These bacteria don't mind acidic conditions, and now that all the other e. coli bacteria are dead, these are free to reproduce, creating more e. coli bacteria that can survive acidic conditions. When these e. coli enter our stomach, they don't always die. Instead, they make us sick.

This is not the only reason to eat grass-fed meat, both farm raised and wild caught. Grass-fed meat is, quite simply, from healthier animals who get fresh air, sunshine, and natural food. They produce a more nutrient dense meat which has more nutrients like omega-3 fatty acids than their industrial counterparts. While vegetable oils and industrial meat lead to an imbalance between omega-3 and omega-6 fatty acids, a diet of healthy fats and grass-fed meat gives us nutrients in the proper ratios.

Small Meat Animals for Homesteaders

Homesteaders who are willing to raise and butcher their own animals have more, and arguably better, options.

All types of fowl—chickens, ducks, turkeys, geese, pheasants—are easy to keep, as are rabbits. They require housing, but a fowl coop or rabbit hutch is much easier and cheaper to build than a barn. They are a smaller investment in money, food, and time. Chickens and rabbits can often be kept even in cities. Small meat animals make a great deal of sense, especially for those who would otherwise have trouble finding affordable, quality meat.

Fish and Seafood

Besides being a prime source for protein, fish like salmon, tuna, anchovies, sardines, herring, and mackerel are also good sources of omega-3 fatty acids. Many people take fish oil supplements to help boost their omega-3 fatty acids. And as I mentioned at the beginning of this chapter, shellfish, liver, fish eggs, octopus, fish, crab, and lobster are all top sources for vitamin B-12.

What Would Cro Think?

Cro would only know about grass-fed meat. If Cro could travel to modern times and visit a CAFO, a Concentrated Animal Feeding Operation, where animals are confined and fed an unnatural diet of grains to make them fat, I think he'd be sad and disgusted. He wouldn't eat those animals either. When he goes out to hunt, he chooses healthy animals. He would know that sick animals aren't healthy to eat.

11

Protein, Part 2

Organ Meats

Do you remember reading about Stefansson and Anderson, the Arctic explorers who ate nothing but meat for a whole year as part of a study? One of the reasons that the men were able to live on nothing but meat without vitamin deficiencies was that they ate the organ meats, too.

Organ meats are some of the most nutrient dense proteins around. They are packed with B vitamins, including the all important B12 that must come from animal sources. Organ meats are also high in minerals like phosphorus, iron, copper, magnesium, iodine, calcium, potassium, sodium, selenium, zinc and manganese. They provide the fat-soluble vitamins A, D, E, and K as well as essential fatty acids.

The liver is one of the mostly widely eaten organ meats. Here in the U. S., liver is eaten from beef, veal, goat, lamb, bison, buffalo, chicken, geese, and duck. Liver is high in vitamin A and the B vitamins. Liver is one of the number top food sources for the mineral copper, and it's also high in folic acid and iron.

Kidneys from beef, lamb and pork are also common. Kidneys are high in the minerals selenium, iron, copper, phosphorus and zinc, and they are particularly high in vitamin B12.

The heart is another top source for the mineral copper, and it is also high in thiamin, folate, selenium, phosphorus, zinc, and many of the B vitamins. Heart also contains twice as much collagen and elastin as regular meat. Collagen and elastin proteins which are particularly good for connective tissue, joint, and digestive health. Connective tissue connects different types of tissue. One of its purposes in the body is to hold organs in place.

When you buy a whole bird, there's often a packet of giblets. Giblets are the organs, and it includes the liver, kidneys, heart, and gizzard. The gizzard is a special type of stomach in some animals like birds which helps to grind up food.

Organ meats should be included in the diet frequently.

Bone Marrow

Bone marrow is another nutrient dense food, so don't give that bone to the dog! Enjoy the marrow yourself. Bone marrow contains protein, calcium, and iron. Bone marrow is also a good source of fat.

When people eat lean meat and leave behind the fat, the organs, and the bone marrow, they're eating the least nutritious parts of an animal. So go wild, and gnaw on a bone.

Pastured Eggs

I considered whether to talk about eggs in the fat chapter or in the protein chapter. Eggs are an excellent source of both. In fact, I believe that eggs may be a perfect food source. Eggs have a moderate amount of protein wrapped around a source of healthy fat.

Another good thing about eggs is that they are relatively inexpensive. People who might not be able to afford high quality meat on a regular basis can often afford high quality eggs daily. Chickens are also easy to keep, and many cities now allow people to keep hens in their backyards.

In our household, we have eggs at both breakfast and lunch on most days. At breakfast, we have eggs in a sugar-free hot cocoa. No, you can't taste the eggs, anymore than you can in ice-cream. But they're there, and they give us a good start to the day. At lunch, we might have boiled, fried, or scrambled eggs. We might have quiche, a kind of egg pie with meat, cheese, and vegetables. We might have green eggs, which are fried eggs with basil pesto and feta cheese.

Eggs are versatile. Add a few ingredients and cook them in

different ways, and you can have eggs quite frequently without getting tired of them.

But what are pastured eggs? Pastured eggs are eggs from hens who are outside, getting plenty of sunlight and able to eat grass and bugs. Chickens who live as Nature intended produce nutrient dense eggs. That means that their eggs have more nutrients than eggs from chickens who are kept in poor conditions. Remember, real food is produced in safe, natural environments.

It shouldn't surprise us that healthy animals produce healthier food. Pastured eggs are known to have more of vitamins A, D, and E. They also have more omega-3 fatty acids and beta carotene. These are real eggs from real chickens, and you can tell the difference. A real egg has a bright orange yolk that stands firm instead of a wimpy, pale yellow yolk that falls apart easily.

Sadly, most stores don't sell real eggs. Remember how organic is mostly a legal term? So are phrases like free-range and cage-free. Legally, a carton of eggs can have these labels even if the chickens who laid the eggs were never able to be outside in the sunshine in their entire lives.

If you can't have chickens in your area, or if your mother said, "No," look for a local farmer who sells pastured eggs. And if you can't get pastured eggs, any egg is still a good source of protein and fat, and is still a much healthier food choice than many you could make.

What Would Cro Think?

Cro would have been used to eating organ meats and bone marrow. In fact, modern hunter-gatherer cultures show us that organ meats and bone marrow are preferred eating. The lean meats, the ones without much fat, are not popular. They're sometimes even thrown out when there's plenty of food (Nicholson). There's a good chance that Cro argued with his little sister over who got the last of the bone marrow.

12

Lacto-Fermented Foods and Bone Broths

Lacto-fermented foods and bone broths are traditionally prepared foods which are so nutritious that they are often called superfoods.

Lacto-Fermented Foods

Unlike other methods of preserving foods, fermenting foods actually makes them more nutritious. Fermenting foods relies on beneficial microbes. When we eat foods with these good microbes, they colonize our gut by reproducing, and they help us to digest our food. Did you know that a healthy human gut has more bacterial cells than human cells? Fermented foods keep our guts healthy.

When foods are fermented, good bacteria eat the sugars and starches in the food. This creates lactic acid, which preserves the food. The process also creates beneficial enzymes, B vitamins, omega-3 fatty acids, and various strains of probiotics.

It sounds odd to rely on microbes to protect us from other microbes. So why is fermentation safe? In the article "Cultivating Their Fascination with Fermentation" by Tara Duggan, Fred Breidt explains:

"With fermented products there is no safety concern. I can flat-out say that. The reason is the lactic acid bacteria that carry out the fermentation are the world's best killers of other bacteria," says Breidt, who works at a lab at North Carolina State University, Raleigh, where scientists have been studying fermented and other pickled foods since the 1930s.

Fermentation is safe because it has the toughest microbes.

Fermented foods have a distinctive sour taste. Pickles and sauerkraut are traditional fermented foods, as are dairy products like yogurt and kefir. Sadly, though, when you find these foods in the grocery store, they are not always truly fermented foods. We say that fermented foods are living because they have live microbes in them. However, many yogurts on the market no longer have active, living cultures of microbes in them. Sauerkrauts are canned using high heat, which kills any microbes that they had. And pickles are often produced by putting cucumbers in vinegar to give them a sour taste.

Like most foods, if you want healthy fermented foods, you'll probably need to make them yourself. There are a couple of books on fermenting foods in the Recommended Reading section at the end of this book.

Bone Broth

Bone broth is a mineral rich liquid made from boiling the bones of an animal. Talk about using the whole animal! Vegetables and herbs are also sometimes added. You can drink the broth alone, salted to taste. It can also be used as a soup base, or it can be used in other recipes in place of liquids such as water. Bone broth is used around the world as an inexpensive, nutrient dense food.

Bone broth is high in calcium, magnesium, and phosphorus. All of these minerals are good for your bones, and your teeth, too. Bone broth also contains collagen and gelatin, which comes from collagen. Collagen is a protein that's good for the health of your joints, hair, skin and nails. Gelatin supports digestive health.

Bone broth is also high in the amino acids glycine and proline. Glycine supports digestion. It also helps the body deal with toxins, which are poisons, and it helps the body to make hemoglobin, which is the protein in red blood cells which carries oxygen to the cells. Proline helps the blood vessels to release cholesterol build-ups, and it helps the body to break down proteins for creating healthy muscle cells. Proline also supports good skin health.

Glycine and proline are not considered essential amino acids. When we say essential in this sense, it means that our bodies cannot produce them. Our bodies can produce glycine and proline. However, it's always better if we can supply our bodies with necessary building blocks.

What Would Cro Think?

While these foods are known to be eaten around the world by traditional cultures, I've not heard of hunter-gatherer cultures using these techniques. I wouldn't be surprised to learn that they did make bone broth, though, because hunter-gatherers are good about finding ways to use the whole animal for food. As for lacto-fermented foods, I think once he got used to the sour flavor, Cro would have appreciated both the taste and the health benefits.

13

Dairy

Dairy is a controversial subject among people who eat in a primal/paleo way. That means that people argue about it. Purists—people who try to eat as closely as possible to the way that people ate during the Paleolithic Era—argue that the domestication of animals began in the Neolithic Era along with farming, so we should avoid dairy. In addition, milk does raise insulin levels. Others argue that people became herder-gatherers before farming, so dairy is okay.

I believe that looking at what people ate prior to agriculture gives us a good set of guidelines, but that doesn't mean that all foods newer than the Paleolithic Era are bad. We should note that dairy products are not necessary for life or good health. This is one of those areas where we each have to look at the facts and decide whether or not the benefits of a food make the bad parts worth it.

However, the dairy in most grocery stores isn't real milk. Like the cows raised for meat, milk cows are not raised in a healthy environment, nor a very clean one. Milk from these big dairies must be pasteurized to be safe. Pasteurization is when they heat milk to a high heat to kill any germs. But when the milk is heated that much, it also kills all of the enzymes. We call unpasteurized milk raw milk since it hasn't been cooked.

The true purpose of milk is to feed baby mammals. Milk contains enzymes to help baby mammals digest the milk. The enzymes can also help us to digest the lactose in milk. Lactose is the sugar that occurs naturally in milk. Many people are lactose intolerant, which means that means that their bodies can't properly digest lactose. With the enzymes in raw milk, though, some people who are lactose intolerant can drink raw milk.

Besides pasteurization, industrial milk goes through another process called homogenization. Normally, the cream in milk separates from the milk and rises to the top; it can be shaken to mix it up again before using it. When milk is homogenized, the cream and milk can't be separated again.

Real milk is produced from cows and goats getting plenty of exercise and sunshine and eating a natural diet of grass. It's produced in a clean and safe environment, so it doesn't have to be pasteurized to be safe. In fact, many people believe that as long as the cow is raised in a healthy environment, the natural lactic-acid producing bacteria in the milk can protect the milk from dangerous bacteria that could cause illness.

Cheese, yogurt, and kefir are products that came from the need to preserve milk. In all three products, good bacteria are added to the milk. The bacteria reproduce and change the milk into a whole new product. These bacteria eat the carbohydrates in milk. Carbohydrates in milk come from the lactose, the milk sugar, so these products are lower in both carbohydrates and lactose than plain milk is. The bacteria in yogurt and kefir are even good for us, as we discussed in the last chapter.

Just as with grass-fed meat and pastured eggs, real milk is more nutrient dense, and the nutrients are more balanced. Dairy is a beneficial part of the diet for many people. However, some people cannot tolerate milk in the diet.

How can you tell if milk is bad for you? Don't have any dairy products for one month, then start using them again, one at a time. If you don't feel as well while having dairy, you shouldn't have dairy.

What Would Cro Think?

We'd all like to know what Cro would think about this subject. Could Cro have been part of a group who kept herds of animals and milked some of them? I think Cro probably would have drank milk, as long as it didn't make him feel bad when he did. But I don't think he would have had it often. After all, Cro may have had milk, but he didn't have a refrigerator!

14

Sweeteners

Sugar is not healthy. It does not matter how natural of a sugar you use; the purest honey on the planet is still bad for you. Sugar is pure carbohydrate, so the problems that come from a high carbohydrate diet are present in a high sugar diet as well. That doesn't mean that you should never have any sort of sugar at all, but it does mean that sugar should be a rare treat, and not something you eat every day.

Do you know what an addiction is? You usually hear that term in connection to drugs; people become addicted to cigarettes as well as many illegal drugs. An addiction is when your body craves a certain substance and feels bad without it.

Did you know that people can be addicted to sugar, too? When you eat a lot of sugar, or a diet high in carbohydrates, your blood sugar is affected. After eating a high carbohydrate meal, blood sugar goes up way higher than it should be as the food is broken down into glucose and sent into the bloodstream. Your body sends out insulin to take care of the excess sugar and stores it as fat. Your blood sugar then falls, or crashes, going way lower than it should be, and your body sends out cravings, a desire to eat something sweet or high in simple carbohydrates, to bring the blood sugar back into a normal range. This is how sugar addiction acts out in the body.

So how do you make your blood sugar normal and stop the blood sugar roller coaster? This question has a simple answer, but it can be hard to do: Quit eating so many carbohydrates and sugar. It's hard to do at first because when your body craves something, even something that's bad for you, you feel bad if you don't have it. People who stop eating sugar may feel tired and cranky for a while.

But the body adjusts quickly. After a few days or a week, the body gets used to using fats and protein for energy. When this happens, blood sugar becomes normal. You have energy without blood sugar crashes and cravings for junk. You start to become healthy. If you are overweight, then you'll also begin to lose weight.

Anytime you have a lot of sugar, you are likely to have a blood sugar crash which makes you crave more. This is why it's not good to have sugar very often.

Tips for Breaking the Sugar Addiction

It is probably best to do away with sweeteners completely except for rare treats. Drink water, and don't sweeten foods. However, sometimes we want something sweet. What do we do then?

There are many artificial sweeteners that people use to replace sugar. They have no sugar, no carbohydrates, so they don't cause problems with blood sugar. However, they also don't fit the primal model. The primal model includes foods that have been part of the diets of healthy people for a long time. Artificial sweeteners are still very new. This is important because it will be a long time before we are able to determine whether or not artificial sweeteners are safe for long term use. Although the government recognizes them as safe, many people, including doctors, already question their safety.

There is a sweetener that is natural and has no carbohydrates. It's a plant called stevia, which means "sweet leaf." It's been used safely for more than 1,500 years by the Guarani people of South America. In Paraguay and Brazil, it has a long history as both a medicinal plant and a sweetener. Stevia is hundreds of times sweeter than sugar: ½ to 1 teaspoon of stevia is equal in sweetness to one cup of sugar.

One problem with stevia is that it can have a bitter aftertaste, and some brands of stevia are worse than others. However, people can adjust to the taste of stevia. Some children who already have a low sugar diet may not have to adjust to it at all. If you do need to, you can do it in about three weeks while getting the sugar out of your diet:

Week 1. Add ½ teaspoon of stevia to one cup of sugar. Use this like you normally use sugar in drinks, but use about ¼ less than normal. That means if you normally use one cup of sugar in a gallon of tea or other type of drink, you'd use ¾ of a cup.

Week 2. Add 1 teaspoon of stevia to one cup of sugar. Use this like you normally use sugar in drinks, but use about ½ less than normal. That means if you normally use one cup of sugar in a gallon of tea or other type of drink, you'd use ½ of a cup.

Week 3. Add 2 teaspoons of stevia to one cup of sugar. Use this like you normally use sugar in drinks, but use about ¾ less than normal. That means if you normally use one cup of sugar in a gallon of tea or other type of drink, you'd use ¼ of a cup of this mixture.

You may notice an aftertaste with each of these steps. It should begin to taste normal to you before going on to the next step.

After this, try stevia plain. Use about ½ to 1 teaspoon to replace a cup of sugar in drinks. To sweeten a cup of tea, it takes just a tiny pinch. Try a smaller amount first, and add more if necessary. Too much stevia can make a drink too sweet and can increase the bitter aftertaste.

Baked Goods

When we bake, sugar does more than just sweeten our food. It also adds volume and texture to our baked goods. That's why when it comes to baking, stevia just isn't enough.

Does this mean we should do away with all baked goods? Not necessarily. Most of us don't bake cakes and cookies every day, anyway. Some people might choose to splurge and have a rare sugar treat, maybe using honey, maple syrup, or another more natural sweetener. I've found that most recipes can easily halve the amount of sugar and still taste great. You can also replace part of the sugar in a recipe with stevia, just not all.

Other people may choose a lower carbohydrate solution, particularly people who have problems with sugar. The most natural low carbohydrate replacement we have are sugar alcohols such as erythritol or xylitol. These are low carbohydrate because the body does not completely absorb them. Because of this, they sometimes cause gas or diarrhea, especially if you eat too much. It's wise to keep the serving size small until you know how these sweeteners affect you.

Chocolate

Primal people like chocolate, too. But did you know that the candy bars in stores are mostly sugar, not chocolate? If you look at the label, sugar is the first ingredient. That means that there's more sugar than any other ingredient.

There are chocolate bars that are mostly chocolate, though. They are called dark chocolate, and they can have anywhere from 70-90% chocolate, with just a touch of sugar. If you like the taste of chocolate, not just sugar, then these bars can give you a treat without causing your blood sugar to spike. They can also be used in a fine chocolate chip cookie, which you can see in the recipe section at the end of this book.

What Would Cro Think?

I bet when Cro came across a bee hive, he enjoyed a little honey. It's natural for humans to enjoy sweet foods. The difference between us and Cro is that he wouldn't have run across a bee hive very often, but we can buy all sorts of sugar at the grocery store every day. If we take our cue from Cro, though, we'll just have a little every once in a while.

15

What are Anti-Nutrients?

Some foods contain substances known as anti-nutrients. Anti means against or opposed to. We call them anti-nutrients because they actually harm the body instead of keeping it healthy. The main foods which contain these anti-nutrients are grains and legumes.

You should remember grains from the original food pyramid. Grains—the bread, cereal, rice, and pasta group—form the base of the pyramid, the group from which the government says you should eat the most. Grains are grass babies, the seeds of certain types of grasses, called cereal grasses. Grains include such foods as wheat, spelt, rye, barley, corn, oats, sorghum, millet, and rice. People commonly eat these grains in a variety of ways, including ground into flour to make things like bread and pasta.

Legumes are pods such as that of peas or beans. Peas, lentils, peanuts, and all types of beans, including soy, are legumes.

There are three main anti-nutrients that grains and legumes have in common: phytic acid, enzyme inhibitors, and lectins.

Phytic Acid

Phytic acid binds itself to minerals like zinc, magnesium, calcium, iron, copper, and others. That means that the minerals become attached, or glued, to the phytic acid. Once the minerals are stuck to the phytic acid, the body can't absorb and use them. The phytic acid robs the body of minerals.

Animals such as cattle, sheep, goats, and deer produce phytase, an enzyme which releases the minerals from the phytic acid for the body's use, so they can eat grasses without any problems. People do not produce phytase, though, so eating lots of foods with phytic acid can lead to mineral deficiencies. A mineral deficiency is when we don't get enough of a mineral, and mineral deficiencies can cause problems such as tooth decay. Remember the Hardin Village farmers? Their grain and legume heavy diet led to malnutrition, shorter lives, more cavities, and more infectious diseases.

Enzyme Inhibitors

An enzyme inhibitor is a molecule that binds to an enzyme and prevents it from working properly.

Grains and legumes are the seeds necessary to produce new plants, and these seeds need certain conditions to begin to grow into new plants. If they start to grow too soon, when it's too cold or too hot, too wet or too dry, then the new plant will die. Because of this, they have enzyme inhibitors that make sure they don't start to grow a new plant until it's safe. This is good for the plant. Unfortunately, our bodies use enzymes to digest our food, so these enzyme inhibitors can stop our bodies from digesting grains and legumes properly. If we can't fully digest these foods, then we can't fully retrieve the nutrients they possess.

Lectins

Lectins are proteins which bind to sugar. Lectins can be found in almost all plants and animals, but they're found in grains and legumes, especially soy, in the highest concentrations. Lectins are very sticky, and because of this, they can bind to the lining—the inside layer—of the small intestine. This leaves the body less able to absorb nutrients. Lectins can also punch tiny holes in the intestinal lining which allows lectins, partially digested food, and toxins to leak into the bloodstream.

When these lectins and food leak into the bloodstream, the body sees them as foreign invaders, and it sends out antibodies. Antibodies lock onto antigens—potentially harmful microbes—and tag them so that another part of the immune system—T cells—can find and destroy them. Unfortunately, sometimes parts of the body look like lectins to the antibodies, and the body begins to attack itself.

The Problem of Gluten

Gluten is a protein found in certain grains. Wheat, spelt, kamut, rye, and barley are some of the most common gluten containing grains.

You may have heard the terms celiac, gluten-intolerance, or gluten-sensitivity. Symptoms can vary from person to person, but can include constipation, diarrhea, bloating, joint pain, and malnourishment. In the most extreme cases—celiac disease—gluten triggers an immune response. That means the body treats gluten as an enemy invader. Antibodies produced in response to gluten flatten the villi in the intestines. The villi are the tiny finger-like projections in the intestines that soak up nutrients from food, absorbing the nutrients as the food travels through the digestive system. When the villi are flattened, they cannot soak up these nutrients, so a person with celiac disease who keeps eating gluten can become malnourished—they don't get all the nutrients they need. People without flattened villi can also have reactions to gluten, even some people who used to be able to eat gluten without any apparent problems.

There are a number of problems with gluten.

First, experts believe that many people are sensitive to gluten but don't realize it. Their symptoms may be mild, and they may have lived with these symptoms for so long that they believe them to be normal.

Second, today's grain has far more gluten it than it did just a hundred years ago. The process that has increased grain yields—how much grain can be produced on a certain amount of land—has also increased the amount of gluten and anti-nutrients.

Third, some people apparently develop celiac disease over time—they're not simply born with it.

For some of us, there's no decision to be made. Gluten damages our bodies in very real, observable ways. For everyone else, it does seem like we don't know all that we need to know about gluten to make an informed decision about including it in our diets.

What Would Cro Think?

Cro wouldn't have had easy access to grains. Maybe he came across them occasionally, and he ate a little. But having access to large amounts of grains requires agriculture, so he never had much. Since he didn't have them often, Cro may have discovered very easily that he didn't feel as well when he ate grains. He might have noticed an upset stomach, or that he felt tired after he ate them.

16

Are Grains and Legumes All Bad All the Time?

Many of the traditional cultures studied by Dr. Weston A. Price in the 1930s ate grains, and yet they did not have the problems that we have with health, obesity, and cavities. If grains are bad, how can this be?

Remember that cereal grains are really grass babies. The purpose of making seeds is reproduction—producing more cereal grasses. Seeds that are fully digested are destroyed; they cannot produce more cereal grasses. Anti-nutrients prevent grains from being digested properly. Animals which eat, but don't completely digest, cereal grasses will then deposit some of the seeds whole in a pile of fertilizer, also known as poop.

In the past, and in more modern traditional cultures, we had vastly different methods of storing and harvesting grain crops. Because crops were harvested by hand, it took longer, allowing the grain to sit in the field for a few days while absorbing rain and dew. This would begin the sprouting process—the process of the seed becoming a new plant. Sprouting decreases the anti-nutrients, as do some ways of preparing grains.

Whole Grains vs. Refined Grains

You may have heard people talk about whole grain and refined grains. What do these terms mean?

Grains are made up of different parts: the germ, the bran, and the

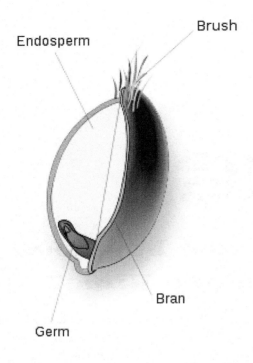

endosperm. Most of the nutritional value in grains—the vitamins, minerals, and fiber—are in the germ and the bran, but these are the parts which are removed to make refined grains. All that's left in refined grains is the endosperm. Manufacturers add some vitamins back to the grain, creating a product that's called enriched.

Refined grains are simple carbohydrates. That means that they're even easier to break down into sugar. They can raise blood sugar faster. Whole grains are complex carbohydrates. They retain the fiber. Fiber can't be digested, so it slows down the digestion of whole grains.

Why would people remove the nutritious part of the plant and eat what's left? There are a couple of reasons. One is taste; many people prefer the taste of refined grains. Another is shelf-life. The bran and germ contain oils that can go rancid. When the bran and germ are removed, the refined grain can be stored for a much longer time before it goes bad.

For the most part, refining grains is helpful only to those who sell grains. However, there may be one exception. In his article "Are Traditionally Prepared Grains Healthy?" Mark Sisson, author of The Primal Blueprint, argued that since the majority of anti-nutrients are removed when rice is refined, refined rice may be the safest grain to eat for people who want to eat grain occasionally.

Preparing Grains and Legumes

Many traditional cultures have developed ways to eat grains and legumes and still maintain good health. None of these methods will remove gluten, but there are some grains such as rice, sorghum, and millet, which are naturally gluten-free. The way they prepare these grains and legumes is the key. Soaking, sprouting, and fermenting are three ways to help reduce phytic acid, enzyme inhibitors, and lectins in grains and legumes.

Soaking and Sprouting

Soaking is simply covering the grains or legumes in water and allowing them to sit for twelve to twenty-four hours in a warm place. Some of the anti-nutrients are water-soluble—they will dissolve in the water. When you pour the water out, some of the anti-nutrients go down the drain with the water.

Sprouting means getting the grains prepared to grow a new plant— that's the sprout. To sprout grains and legumes, first soak them overnight. In the morning, drain the grains or legumes in a colander; rinse them and cover them with a towel. Keep them in the colander, and put the colander in a bowl. This allows the water to keep draining off of them. Rinse them morning and evening for two to four days, until sprouts appear. After that, they can be cooked as usual.

Soaking and sprouting do not reduce phytic acid by much, but they do deactivate many enzyme inhibitors. As for lectins, they are significantly reduced in some foods, but hardly at all in others.

Fermenting

Remember that fermentation uses good bacteria to change our food. When grains are fermented, it can help to reduce anti-nutrients.

Grains have traditionally been mixed with a starter culture or allowed to wild ferment. Starter cultures are types of good bacteria such as those found in whey, kefir, and yogurt. Wild fermentation uses bacteria already on the grains and in the environment.

Fermentation does reduce the amount of anti-nutrients by significant amounts, but the fermentation process can take one to four days to get this result.

One way to use fermented grains is in sourdough bread. Like other fermented foods, sourdough bread has a sour taste.

So What's the Verdict on Grains and Legumes?

Without proper preparation, the anti-nutrients render grains downright dangerous to eat. But even with proper preparation, they are no more nutritious than a diet of meat and vegetables, and they are high in carbohydrate, which causes problems in the body. Proper preparation is also a rather time consuming task that can take a great deal of planning.

Legumes in particular can be a very inexpensive, easy to store source of protein. After all, this is one of the reasons that grains and legumes originally gained popularity. But even though soaking, sprouting, and fermenting do make it easier for us to use the vitamins and minerals in grains and legumes, some of the anti-nutrients still remain.

In the end, these foods take a lot of work for little nutritional benefit. Since there's no sure way to get rid of all of the anti-nutrients, I do not believe that these foods should be a regular part of the diet. However, each family will have to decide for itself whether or not grains and legumes should be included on occasion.

What Would Cro Think?

Would Cro want to add grains and legumes to his diet? He might. They do taste good, and his people could have learned how to properly prepare them. Would he have even known that they might harm his health? Probably not. It's hard to imagine anyone choosing to spend all of that time growing and harvesting food that would make him sick. And during Cro's time, the only way to have grains and legumes regularly would have been to give up his hunter-gatherer lifestyle and become a farmer instead. That would have made the decision easy for Cro. We have to look at other issues, like cost and the ability to store food easily. Are grains and legumes worth it?

17

A Low-Carb Lifestyle

I've seen many people ask whether or not children should be on low-carb diets. A low-carb diet is one that doesn't have many carbohydrates in it. But I have a different question: Why shouldn't children eat a low-carb diet? Remember that carbohydrates are not necessary for life. They are not necessary sources of nutrients or energy.

Some children, through no fault of their own, are more likely to have weight problems. Other children could eat tons of carbohydrates throughout childhood and not have a weight problem until they enter their twenties. Other people never have weight problems from eating carbohydrates, but they do develop health problems—the diseases of civilization—such as heart disease and diabetes. For almost everyone, high-carb diets eventually lead to health or weight problems, or both. So I ask again, since carbohydrates are not necessary, why should anyone eat a lot of them?

On the other hand, I can think of reasons not to eat a lot of carbohydrates. If you start eating low-carb as a child, then you will have a healthy diet from the beginning, one which you can continue to enjoy throughout your entire life. You will not have to change your diet as you get older. This is important because your tastes are formed by what you eat regularly. Also, people who eat a lot of carbohydrates crave more carbohydrates.

Don't misunderstand me, though. We don't count carbohydrates in our household. Instead, we have a steady diet of healthy foods that we all enjoy. We are almost completely sugar-free—we all enjoy a piece of dark chocolate occasionally—and we are mostly grain-free—we have gluten-free pasta or rice about once a month. This alone makes us a low-carb household because sugar and grains are the highest carbohydrate foods.

Vegetables

None of this means that we should never eat carbs. In fact, it would be difficult to have a zero carb diet. It would mean that we could only eat meat and fat. It is possible, as long as the people eating this way eat the whole animal, organs and all. But it's not necessary.

Vegetables have carbs, but not too many carbs. In fact, for most vegetables, it would be hard to eat enough to make your insulin spike.

Vegetables and fruits are also the only source of phytonutrients. Phytonutrients are chemicals in plants which protect the plant from germs, fungi, bugs, and other threats. These phytonutrients also protect our bodies.

Leafy green vegetables like spinach, kale, and collards contain the phytonutrients lutein and zeaxanthin, which are good for eye health.

Fruits such as strawberries, raspberries, and pomegranates contain the phytonutrient ellagic acid, which is believed to help prevent cancer.

Yellow, orange, and red fruits and vegetables contain carotenoids, which are antioxidants.

Vegetables are packed with vitamins, minerals, and antioxidants. Remember that those antioxidants protect the body against free radicals in search of an electron. You should still eat your liver (and heart, and kidneys), but you should eat your veggies, too.

Enjoy in Moderation

There are also a couple of natural, whole foods that can be enjoyed in moderation, even if they're not good for us on a daily basis.

Fruits are technically a paleo whole food. But even though they predate agriculture, that doesn't mean that agriculture hasn't changed them. While berries are a low carbohydrate treat that can be enjoyed often, most other fruits have been specifically grown to be high in sugar. Keep in mind that your body does not care about the source of the sugar; it treats them the same. So, while this tastes good, fruits are not something that we should have all the time. However, as an occasional higher carbohydrate treat, fruit of any variety is a great option.

Potatoes are not allowed on a strict paleo diet, but it must be a rare person who doesn't love the humble spud. As a pure starch, however, they have a high carbohydrate count. It doesn't take many, though. Just a few fried up with some meat and vegetables satisfy. Ironically, the sweet potato actually has fewer carbohydrates than a regular potato, so we feel comfortable having them more often.

Nuts, Berries, and Pork Rinds

What is a primal snack? Primal snacks should be like any other primal food—whole, and filled with healthy fats and proteins.

Nuts and seeds rank high on the list of healthy snacks, with almonds rated first among them. Nuts are high in healthy fats and proteins. They can be enjoyed by the handful, or made into nut butters. Peanuts are actually a legume, not a nut, so they are not a primal food. However, many people find almond butter or sunflower seed butter even better. Almonds, as well as some other nuts, can be ground into a nut meal, like a flour, and used for baked goods. Those who are dairy free by necessity or choice can also use nut milk as a milk substitute.

Berries are the healthiest fruits around. They are low in carbohydrates and high in antioxidants and other nutrients. Berries are packed with vitamin C, and they have other vitamins and minerals as well. There are many varieties of berries: strawberries, blueberries, black berries, raspberries, cranberries, loganberries, currants, gooseberries, lingonberries and bilberries. They can be enjoyed fresh in season. During the rest of the year, many varieties are easy to find frozen. Frozen berries can be added to smoothies, or even added to an almond flour muffin.

Pork rinds are primal chips. They satisfy the urge for something crunchy and salty, and they give an alternative for eating healthy dips, like guacamole.

The truth is, there are plenty of primal snacks. Once we get past the idea that a snack includes a bread product or sugar, we find an abundance of snack ideas. Olives and cheese are full of healthy fats. Green smoothies, with yogurt, spinach, berries, and a touch of stevia, are full of vitamins, leafy greens, and good bacteria. Boiled eggs can be cooked in advance and stored in the refrigerator; they can be eaten with mustard, homemade mayonnaise, or a little salad dressing.

What Would Cro Think?

Cro wouldn't call it low-carb eating. He'd just call it eating. It wouldn't be anything special for him to eat lots of fatty meat with some nuts, berries, and vegetables. Cro would be surprised to hear from people of our time period that good health depends on foods he'd never even heard of. Cro was lean and active. He didn't eat a lot of carbs because he didn't have access to a lot of carbs. And you know what? He was healthier for the lack.

18

Sleep and Play

There's more to good health than just diet.

The body needs plenty of sleep. You probably know that people get cranky when they haven't had enough sleep, but there's more to it than that. The circadian rhythm is a 24 hour cycle of processes that our bodies goes through. But it's not merely an internal rhythm; the circadian rhythm can be affected by outside influences. One of those is light.

People are affected by light. We naturally start waking up when sunlight enters the room, and we naturally get tired when it starts to get dark. These light cues tell our bodies when to produce melatonin. Melatonin is the sleep hormone. Our bodies are naturally geared to be awake during daylight hours, and asleep during the dark hours.

But the word "naturally" doesn't have much to do with how most of us live today. Once it gets dark outside, most Americans still sit in well-lit houses, possibly watching television or using the computer. Household lights, televisions, and computers are all bright blue lights which disrupt our circadian cycles. When those cycles are disrupted—when people don't get enough light during the daytime, or when they get too much at night—melatonin is not produced at the right times, and people have trouble sleeping.

Sleep deprivation—not getting enough sleep—makes it hard for people to concentrate. Lack of sleep can also weaken the immune system, which will cause people to get sick more often. It can lead to stress and medical problems like high blood pressure.

Sleep is especially important for children. Most children need ten to eleven hours of sleep every night. You are growing fast, and your body needs sleep to grow.

The solution is a simple one. When the sun goes down, reduce and eliminate lights around the house. Turn off the screens, both television and computer—anything that's shining blue light right at your face. Turn household lights down low. Some people say that yellow light bulbs do not disrupt circadian rhythms.

Our household is off-grid. That means that we don't get electricity from the electric company. Instead, we have solar panels which charge a battery array that powers our household. We have small rechargeable lights that we use after dark. Each of us also has a head-light, a small flash-light that can be worn on the head, that we use for reading. After dark, we don't have enough power to run bright lights, but we soon realized that this is a blessing. We all sleep better than we used to.

Play

Yes, you need play. This isn't something I can tell you about. Children are the experts when it comes to play, so you should send me a lesson!

When we talk about play in this context, we're mainly talking about physical activity. Children naturally run and jump, rest for a bit, and then start up again. You move a lot, and your mother probably says things like, "I wish I had that kind of energy." But if you play sports, or do other physically demanding activities, your idea of play may be relaxing with a book. The point is to move some, relax some, enjoy life.

You may not realize it, but you already have the beginning of a lifetime of healthy physical activity based in your play. So I'm not saying that this is something you should do. Instead, I'm saying: Don't stop!

Work and Play

You may not realize it, but play is an important part in the lives of modern hunter-gatherers. According to Dr. Peter Gray in his article "Play Makes Us Human," modern hunter-gatherers usually don't even have a word that means the same thing that we mean when we say "work." Dr. Gray writes, "Their own work is simply an extension of children's play. Children play at hunting, gathering, hut construction, tool making, meal preparations, defense against predators, birthing, infant care, healing, negotiation, and so on and so on; and gradually, as their play become increasingly skilled, the activities become productive."

Their daily labor is not unpleasant toil. Instead, they spend the days with their friends and family. They perform tasks that are fun, that vary from day to day, and that require skill and intelligence. There's not a lot of it, and no one has to do it. Doesn't that sound like play?

What Would Cro Think?

Cro got plenty of sleep, plenty of play, and plenty of productive activity to fill his days. Like the diet, I think this is another part of hunter-gatherer culture we'd be wise to pick up and make our own.

A Few Recipes

This is not primarily a recipe book, so there are only a few recipes here. Most of these recipes are family favorites which keep us from having sugar or grain-filled versions of these foods. A couple are just good recipes to have for a low-carb lifestyle.

Cool Aid

Sometimes we want something more than water, but it seems that every flavored water or drink mix that we've found has something wrong with it—sugar, dyes, or maltodextrin, it's always something. Our solution is not perfect, but it's the best we've come up with so far. We use Capella Flavor Drops, which can contain both natural and artificial flavors, with citric acid and a touch of stevia. The fruit flavors are the ones that seem to work best in water.

We make a large container without adding the flavor drops so each person can decide which flavor he wants.

½ gallon water

1 tsp citric acid

¼ tsp stevia

32 drops Capella Flavor Drops

Hot Cocoa

We make hot cocoa every morning for breakfast. This can also be chilled for chocolate milk.

Make sure you cook this thoroughly, especially if you do not trust your eggs to be free from salmonella and other dangerous pathogens. It should cook until it reaches 160° F, or until it thickens and coats the back of a spoon. This means that when I run my finger through the cocoa on the spoon, it leaves a clean path.

For one large serving or two small servings:

2 eggs
1 3/4 cup milk of choice (we use coconut milk)
2 tablespoons cocoa powder
1 teaspoon vanilla
stevia to taste

Cook the nut milk until it just begins to boil. (If using dairy milk, take it off the heat before it gets to boiling.) While mixing the eggs with a whisk or stick blender, slowly pour part of the hot milk into the eggs to temper them. Return the milk and egg mixture to the pot and mix. I check the temperature at this point. It's normally 160 degrees at this point, so the eggs are thoroughly cooked. If it's below 160, I return it to the stove and cook it until it coats the back of a spoon.

Warning: If you cook this on high heat, you run the risk of scorching or curdling it. If this happens, you can salvage it with a stick blender.

Add the stevia and vanilla.

Yogurnut

We heard of a make-ahead breakfast recipe with yogurt and chia seeds. Sadly, when we found an actual recipe, the main ingredient was oatmeal. So, we created our own primal version.

32 ounces full fat yogurt

2½ ounces unsweetened coconut
8 ounces pecan meal (make pecan meal, or the nut meal of your choice, by putting the nuts in a food processor or coffee grinder)
4 tablespoons chia seeds

EITHER ½ teaspoon stevia and ½ cup cocoa powder

OR ¼ teaspoon stevia and 16 ounces berries of choice

Mix all ingredients together and let sit in refrigerator overnight. Place in individual-serving sized jars, if desired, for quick serve breakfasts or snacks.

Chocolate Chip Cookies

These fall to pieces when they're warm, but they're worth eating with a spoon. The tablespoon of molasses means that they're not technically sugar-free, but it could be left out.

4 cups almond flour
1 teaspoon baking soda
1 teaspoon salt

1 cup (2 sticks) butter
5/8 cup erythritol + 5/8 teaspoon stevia OR 5/8 cup of Truvia®
2 tablespoons vanilla
1 tablespoon molasses
1 egg

7 ounces 70% chocolate (We freeze 70% chocolate bars and then smash them with a hammer.)

Preheat oven to 350 for cookies, 325 for cookie bars. Mix the first three dry ingredients.

Cream the butter, erythritol, stevia, vanilla, and molasses together. Add the egg and mix thoroughly. Add the dry mixture. Stir in the chocolate chunks.

Bake cookies for 9-11 minutes. Bake cookie bars for 20-25 minutes.

Coconut Ghee

This cooking fat gives the best properties of both ghee and coconut oil, and it lessens the coconut flavor.

1 pound of unsalted butter
1 pound of unrefined coconut oil

First, use the butter to prepare ghee. Bring butter to a boil over medium-high heat, approximately 2-3 minutes. Reduce heat to medium. A foam will form, but it will disappear. Ghee is done when a second foam appears and the ghee turns golden, approximately 7-8 minutes. The milk solids will be brown and at the bottom of the pan. Pour ghee through a fine mesh strainer or through cheesecloth into a heat-proof container.

The ghee can be left out on the countertop and used as-is for cooking. There are different schools of thought on how long ghee will last unrefrigerated, but the process of making ghee removes the water content and the milk solids—the stuff that goes bad. Like anything, if it smells bad, don't eat it.

To make Tropical Cow, while the ghee is still hot, add an equal amount of coconut oil. Stir, store in an airtight container, and use for any cooking needs.

Cheese Pizza Crust

This feeds our family of seven—barely. This is one of the tastiest gluten-free pizza crusts we've ever tried, and it's certainly the easiest to make.

For a more traditional, though slightly higher-carb crust, we like the recipe in The Zen Belly Cookbook.

For the crust:

8 ounces grated mozzarella
8 ounces grated cheddar

4 eggs

Optional: 8-16 ounces chopped spinach or finely chopped cauliflower

For the toppings:

Approximately 12 ounces spaghetti sauce or pesto
12-16 ounces of mozzarella cheese
Other toppings of choice

Preheat oven to 350-400.

Mix the crust ingredients together. If you use frozen spinach, thaw first in a colander, and press with towels to get the excess liquid out. Bake crust for about 7-10 minutes, until the crust is solid.

Add toppings. Bake for an additional 7-10 minutes.

Quiche

This is our basic quiche recipe. We make two of these to feed our family of seven, though we haven't tried it since our family went dairy milk-free.

6 eggs
1 cup cream
½ cup milk
4 ounces cheese
8 ounces bacon, sausage, or other meat
8 ounces mushrooms or vegetable of choice
¼ teaspoon salt
¼ teaspoon pepper
¼ teaspoon minced dried garlic

We use an 11 inch round pan. Preheat oven to 325. Whisk together eggs, milk, cream, and spices. Add other ingredients. Bake for 35 minutes or until quiche is set.

Bibliography / Recommended Reading and Viewing

For children, I highly recommend The Omnivore's Dilemma: Young Reader's Editon by Michael Pollan. I also highly recommend Fat Head for everyone. Although they don't understand it all, even my youngest children enjoy watching it. The rest of these book suggestions are for adults and teens who are ready for the grown-up versions.

The Complete Idiot's Guide to Fermenting Foods by Wardeh Harmon

Get Your Fats Straight by Sarah Pope

Fat Head, a film by Tom Naughton

The Omnivore's Dilemma: Young Reader's Editon by Michael Pollan

The Omnivore's Dilemma by Michael Pollan

The Primal Blueprint by Mark Sisson

Protein Power by Drs. Eades

Real Food Fermentation: Preserving Whole Fresh Food with Live Cultures in Your Home Kitchen by Alex Lewin

Why We Get Fat And What to Do About It by Gary Taubes

Works Cited

Duggan, Tara. "Cultivating Their Fascination with Fermentation." San Francisco Chronicle 7 June 2009. Web. 25 March 2013.

Fat-Head. Tom Naughton. Morningstar Entertainment, 2009. Film.

Gray, Peter. "Play Makes Us Human V: Why Hunter-Gatherers' Work is Play." Psychology Today 2 July 2009. Web. 13 June 2013.

Nicholson, Ward. "Setting the Scientific Record Straight on Humanity's Evolutionary Prehistoric Diet and Ape Diets." BeyondVeg.com. Beyond Vegetarianism, 24 March 2000. Web. 14 June 2013.

Pope, Sarah. Get Your Fats Straight. 2013. eBook.

Sisson, Mark. "Are Traditionally Prepared Grains Healthy?" Marksdailyapple.com. Mark's Daily Apple, 3 August 2011. Web. 25 March 2013.

Stefansson, Vilhjalmur. "Adventures in Diet." Drbass.com. Life Science International Fasting Center, n.d. Web. 26 June 2013.

Taubes, Gary. Good Calories, Bad Calories. New York: Alfred A. Knopf, 2008. Print.

Made in the USA
Middletown, DE
27 July 2019